# NO SUGAR DIET

## The Only Diet
## that really works!

## DIET GUIDLINES
## PLUS 4 WEEK DIET JOURNAL

### BY

Denise Blair

Denise Blair is an author of several Christian books (devotionals, prayer books, No Sugar Diet Pledge and many others).

DISCLAIMER: The contents of this book are provided for general informational purposes. This material is not meant to substitute the advice provided by a medical healthcare professional. This information is not intended to diagnose or treat medical conditions or substitute appropriate medical care. If you are under the care of a physician and take medications for diabetes, heart disease, high blood pressure or any other medications, consult your healthcare provider prior to engaging in any diet program. Author hereby wishes to better the health of all who are caught up in the repetitious cycle of sugar addiction; however, makes no claims to the written material here. It is the responsibility of the individual(s) reading this material to work with his/her physician and to have cholesterol and lipid profiles done before during and after initiating any diet. Author only attests to the health saving benefits that she encountered by abstaining from refined sugar. Author thereby is not held responsible for any adverse outcome to following this diet – and sincerely advises working with your healthcare provider. If you are significantly overweight – please be under the care of a physician. Blood pressure medications may need to be reduced when adhering to this diet – as this diet with the elimination of sugar brings down blood sugar and blood pressure levels while reducing weight and hunger.

Sugar, sugar – everywhere – no store, isle or convenient store with shortage to spare.

Sugar – it is everywhere you go – in each store, gas station and convenient store. Pop out of the fountains, candy bars by the register, grab and go snacks throughout the store. Sugar is only adding to an already overweight population, diabetes, health disease, and many other kinds of problems.

You don't have to be a slave to the addiction of sugar – which is highly addictive. One bite leads to another. Just say "no" to sugar and get off the roller coaster highs and lows of sugar addiction.

I lost weight by eating fat and protein. The low fat diet craze only made me gain weight, crave sugar and added cellulite to my body. I went through extreme withdrawals from sugar – sort of like getting off a very addictive drug. Insomnia, anxiety, bad dreams and more were part of my withdrawal symptoms. I was also diagnosed with a fatty liver prior to removing all sugar from my diet. Sugar is broken down into triglycerides and excess triglycerides are stored as fat on hips and thighs and in the liver and other organs.

I now have palmar erythema – indicative of liver damage. You can reverse this addiction and damage to your body and regain a youthful figure, if you start today – by avoiding refined sugar.

Refined sugar also causes hyperactivity and mood disorders (ADD, depression, anxiety).

## SUGAR ADDICTION

Do you have trouble losing weight and keeping it off? Do you have trouble with an appetite that won't quit? What about your energy – do you have the energy you desire? Concentration you desire? The health and wellbeing you desire? Having too much sugar in your diet – or any at all, – wrecks havoc on your health and can and does make for an ill temperament. Do you have trouble avoiding those sugary drinks and other fast food grabs at the check-out? You are not alone with your sugar addiction.

The ills of overweight people and people who cannot lose weight effectively, in my opinion, is due to refined sugar and carbohydrate in the diet. We were not designed to eat processed high in sugar snacks and drinks. The ills of Americans can be traced to processed sugar and manufactured foods and drinks loaded with it. A single soda – a small can contains 7-8 teaspoons of sugar – more than you should get in an entire day. Your blood sugar goes up and then drops and you reach for another high in sugar snack or soft drink. And the cycle continues.

Sugar addiction is real – sugar is killing Americans. We are an eat on the run nation – grabbing things at the check-out, out of the vending machines and gobbling our way to obesity at staggering rates.

Our bodies are not designed for sugar. We are designed for natural foods – proteins, vegetables, fruits and grains. Sugar robs you of your health, sanity and productivity. Eventually it will rob you of your life.

Sugar sets the stage for other addictions: alcohol, tobacco, prescription meds and illegal drugs. Sugar is known to cause hyperactivity, ADD, weight gain, mood swings, cardiovascular disease and much more. You can stop the addiction; you can regain control of your life, your health and overweight problems.

If you get the sugar out of your diet – you will reduce your appetite as your blood sugar levels return to normal. You will reduce anxiety and think more clearly and rationally. There are many other benefits to getting the sugar out – being sugar-free for life. You can improve cardiovascular health, reduce weight and have smoother skin (getting rid of cellulite). You will regain new energy and freedom from thinking about that next meal or snack. Refined sugar just sets the stage for disaster. It is time to get the sugar out of the diets of Americans.

First – clean out the cupboards – throw out the refined, packaged, sweetened foods (cereal, cookies, pop, ice cream and other so called goodies).

Next – make a trip to the store and stock up on meats (protein), cheese, vegetables and some fruits. The outer isles of your grocery store are where you want to spend your time and money.

God didn't design our bodies for sugar. He designed us for natural foods – proteins, vegetables, fruits and grains. He didn't design us to consume manufactured highly addictive sugary products.

God gave us dominion over the livestock, over every creature on this earth, over every herb bearing seed. He didn't say go out and refine all these things and produce unnatural sugar sweetened foods and drinks. America was a relatively thin society (pre 1980's) before the so-called low fat diet was thrown at us and all the manufacturing plants that popped up producing high in sugar and calorie snacks. Before 1980, you didn't have refrigerated cooler after cooler in the stores loaded with soft drinks, sports drinks and sweetened coffee and energy drinks. You didn't have bakeries in each and every big box store. You didn't have isle after isle of cookies, snack cakes and other sweet snacks. Obesity and diet was not the ongoing news that it is today. In the 80's, you didn't have 20 different antidepressants on the market. My feeling in many cases – that sugar causes anxiety as well as depression – but a psychiatrist will find another reason for it.  I've been there too – done that – nothing worked until I got my diet (removing all refined sugar) under control. I think there is a connection to the sugar society we have become and popping pills – pills for diabetes, pills for cholesterol, pills for blood pressure, pills for anxiety and the list goes on. And even the drug use/addiction in young teens and adults.

If you get the refined sugar out of your diet – you will actually reduce your appetite as your blood sugar levels return to normal. Anxiety, hypertension, depression will disappear. Increased energy and clear thinking will become part of your no sugar diet. Your weight will gradually reduce – it won't happen overnight – you didn't put it on in a month or two – it will gradually reduce.

You can improve cardiovascular health; get rid of cellulite or that spare tire. Sleep will become more peaceful. Refined sugar just sets the stage for disaster – it is time to get the sugar out. Withdrawals from sugar are real. Prepare ahead of time by stocking up on healthy protein foods – meats, fish, chicken, cheese, vegetables, eggs, cottage cheese and nuts.  You may experience a headache for a few days, you might feel flu-like, you may have trouble sleeping – these are all withdrawals symptoms from refined sugar.

You will lose a lot of water on this diet as sugar causes water retention.  So you will need to have bottled water or diet drinks on hand to rehydrate.

My withdrawals from sugar included:

1. Depression
2. Anxiety
3. Cravings for sweets
4. Tremors in my hands
5. Feelings of bugs on the walls
6. Insomnia and bad dreams
7. Fatigue – for the first week
8. Extreme loss of water
9. Extreme thirst
10. Flashbacks of things in my life – like an alcoholic might have flashbacks
11. Low blood sugar and the need to eat as my blood sugar plummeted with removing refined sugar
12. Itching of my skin
13. Feeling flu-like for a week

Be prepared to not feel very well for several days.  The weekend might be a good time to start – if you work out of the home.  Make a promise to yourself – to never reach for the sweetened coffee, donut or ice cream again.

HERE'S THE PLAN –

Avoid refined sugar, sweets, limit starches and weight loss will begin. In a short time you will see weight loss, cellulite disappear and find renewed energy and health and a better outlook on life. It may take several days or a couple of weeks to feel better/stable.

LET'S BEGIN:

1. We begin the diet by stopping/removing all sweets from the diet. Throw them out, stop wasting money and health on sugary drinks, pops, so called energy drinks, coffee laced with sugar, donuts, etc. Sugar is poison – stop buying packaged cookies, store bought pies and junk in a box items. No candy in any form – chocolate, ice cream must go. Yogurt is laced with sugar. Unfortunately alcohol is full of empty calories and is broken down into sugar that you will store as fat.

2. Think protein foods – eggs, meat, chicken and fish. Have some dairy (milk, cheese, eggs), some fruits, vegetables and some starch (bread, rice, pasta). These are the main foods

on a no sugar diet.  The meat portion should be the largest item on your plate, then a vegetable and a fruit or a starch.  Think fist sized portions.

3.   Dessert if you must should consist of fruit and cheese or nuts.

4.  You can eat satisfying food on this diet.  You will regain control of your appetite.


Allowed foods:

Meats – a fist sized portion at each meal (3 meals a day).  Meats include beef, ham, chicken, pork, turkey, sausage, fish, seafood, lamb, bacon.  You can grill, fry, or roast – any way you like.

Cheese – it is good to have cheese and crackers on hand – when you feel the urge to nibble/snack.

Eggs – any and cooked any style.  1-2 eggs each morning for breakfast.  Egg salad is good in the summertime.  Or have a hardboiled egg with cheese, or poached or deviled eggs are also good.

Milk is allowed – a cup of whole milk at each meal if desired.

Butter – is not the bad guy here.

Potatoes: in moderation, a serving the size of a closed fist is enough. Choose other vegetables with your meals or choose potatoes every other day.

Vegetables: Most vegetables are low in starch. Try to have a serving with each meal.

Fruit: as a dessert or with cheese – ½ an apple, a hand full of grapes is enough.

Starch: rice, pasta, noodles – limit to ½-1 cup per meal.

Break/toast/bun: 1 slice per meal.

Try to keep your complex carb intake (fruits, vegetables, bread and potatoes) to less than 120 grams a day. You will lose weight steadily and at a pace that is healthy.

Menu:

Breakfast: 1-2 eggs anyway you like. If you don't like eggs – have cottage cheese and a slice of toast. You could have a breakfast sandwich, a hash brown or sausage gravy and 2 biscuits. ½ cup of orange juice is enough or ½ a banana.

Lunch: The list is endless. BLT, egg salad sandwich, steak sandwich, hamburger, ham sandwich, steak, chicken. Just pick a protein source first, then a starch (1-2 slices bread, 1 roll or 1 bun). If you like salads – they are low in starch – but have some protein with it. You do not have to restrict mayo or butter. Have a little salad with half a sandwich or Cole Slaw if you want to reduce the bread in your diet. ½ a piece of fruit such as an apple or an orange is enough. You could have apple sauce without sugar or a few potato chips or a small order of fries. Just remember you are aiming for less than 120 grams of carbohydrate a day.

Dinner: You will need to spend a little time in the kitchen and prepare ahead of time, so you will have something in the fridge when you are tempted to snack. Make dinners ahead of time; spaghetti, lasagna, stuffed cabbage, chicken breasts and steak. Dinner should consist of a protein portion first (a first sized serving), a vegetable (a cup is enough), a starch such as noodles, rice or pasta (about a cup or less).

Try to think of your plate as a pie – a small pie – and 1/3 of that should be your protein source, 1/3 should be your vegetable and 1/3 your starch. Add a roll or slice of garlic toast – maybe just not every night.

For dessert or snacks – have cheese and crackers, ½ a piece of fruit or nuts.

Learn to read labels for carb and sugar content. Aim for less that 120 grams of carbs a day – and avoid any and all sugary snacks.

---

# 4 WEEK LOW CARB/ NO SUGAR DIET JOURNAL

Use the 4 week diet journal – to train yourself to keeping your carb intake at levels that only satisfy your diet and sustain your health.  After 4 weeks of keeping track – it should become second nature without having to think too much about avoiding sweets and keeping carb intake low.

Date/Day #1:_____

Protein:  0 0 0 0  - Up to 4 fist sized portions a day.  Fill in each circle as you choose/eat your protein source.

Dairy:  0 0 0 – Milk or cheese – ½-1 cup of milk at each meal or slice of cheese.

Carbs:  0 0 0 – This includes your rice, noodles, pasta and bread.  ½ - 1 cup is enough 1-2 times a day.  Bread – a slice or one bun two times a day.

Fruit:  0 0 - Each serving of fruit should be equal to ½ apple or hand full of grapes.

Veg:  0 0 0 0 – choose low in carb vegetables – which most vegetables are except potatoes, yams and sweet potatoes.

Water/ diet drinks – you will need to replace the liquid you lose on this diet.  Drink what you need to replace that and stay hydrated.

Try to think of portion sizes equal to a closed fist and try to remember the pie plate technique – first a protein (a third of your plate), then a vegetable and then a starch.

Fill in the circles as you choose the right foods for weight loss.

Date/Day #2:_____

Protein:  0 0 0 0  - Up to 4 fist sized portions a day.  Fill in each circle as you choose/eat your protein source.

Dairy:  0 0 0 – Milk or cheese – ½-1 cup of milk at each meal or slice of cheese.

Carbs:  0 0 0 – This includes your rice, noodles, pasta and bread.  ½ - 1 cup is enough 1-2 times a day.  Bread – a slice or one bun two times a day.

Fruit:  0 0 - Each serving of fruit should be equal to ½ apple or hand full of grapes.

Veg:  0 0 0 0 – choose low in carb vegetables – which most vegetables are except potatoes, yams and sweet potatoes.

Water/ diet drinks – you will need to replace the liquid you lose on this diet.  Drink what you need to replace that and stay hydrated.

Try to think of portion sizes equal to a closed fist and try to remember the pie plate technique – first a protein (a third of your plate), then a vegetable and then a starch.

Fill in the circles as you choose the right foods for weight loss.

Date/Day #3:_____

Protein:  0 0 0 0  - Up to 4 fist sized portions a day.  Fill in each circle as you choose/eat your protein source.

Dairy:  0 0 0 – Milk or cheese – ½-1 cup of milk at each meal or slice of cheese.

Carbs:  0 0 0 – This includes your rice, noodles, pasta and bread.  ½ - 1 cup is enough 1-2 times a day.  Bread – a slice or one bun two times a day.

Fruit:  0 0 - Each serving of fruit should be equal to ½ apple or hand full of grapes.

Veg:  0 0 0 0 – choose low in carb vegetables – which most vegetables are except potatoes, yams and sweet potatoes.

Water/ diet drinks – you will need to replace the liquid you lose on this diet.  Drink what you need to replace that and stay hydrated.

Try to think of portion sizes equal to a closed fist and try to remember the pie plate technique – first a protein (a third of your plate), then a vegetable and then a starch.

Fill in the circles as you choose the right foods for weight loss.

Date/Day #4:_____

Protein:  0 0 0 0  - Up to 4 fist sized portions a day.  Fill in each circle as you choose/eat your protein source.

Dairy:  0 0 0 – Milk or cheese – ½-1 cup of milk at each meal or slice of cheese.

Carbs:  0 0 0 – This includes your rice, noodles, pasta and bread.  ½ - 1 cup is enough 1-2 times a day.  Bread – a slice or one bun two times a day.

Fruit:  0 0 - Each serving of fruit should be equal to ½ apple or hand full of grapes.

Veg:  0 0 0 0 – choose low in carb vegetables – which most vegetables are except potatoes, yams and sweet potatoes.

Water/ diet drinks – you will need to replace the liquid you lose on this diet.  Drink what you need to replace that and stay hydrated.

Try to think of portion sizes equal to a closed fist and try to remember the pie plate technique – first a protein (a third of your plate), then a vegetable and then a starch.

Fill in the circles as you choose the right foods for weight loss.

Date/Day #5:_____

Protein:  0 0 0 0  - Up to 4 fist sized portions a day.  Fill in each circle as you choose/eat your protein source.

Dairy:  0 0 0 – Milk or cheese – ½-1 cup of milk at each meal or slice of cheese.

Carbs:  0 0 0 – This includes your rice, noodles, pasta and bread.  ½ - 1 cup is enough 1-2 times a day.  Bread – a slice or one bun two times a day.

Fruit:  0 0 - Each serving of fruit should be equal to ½ apple or hand full of grapes.

Veg:  0 0 0 0 – choose low in carb vegetables – which most vegetables are except potatoes, yams and sweet potatoes.

Water/ diet drinks – you will need to replace the liquid you lose on this diet.  Drink what you need to replace that and stay hydrated.

Try to think of portion sizes equal to a closed fist and try to remember the pie plate technique – first a protein (a third of your plate), then a vegetable and then a starch.

Fill in the circles as you choose the right foods for weight loss.

Date/Day #6:_____

Protein:  0 0 0 0  - Up to 4 fist sized portions a day.  Fill in each circle as you choose/eat your protein source.

Dairy:  0 0 0 – Milk or cheese – ½-1 cup of milk at each meal or slice of cheese.

Carbs:  0 0 0 – This includes your rice, noodles, pasta and bread.  ½ - 1 cup is enough 1-2 times a day.  Bread – a slice or one bun two times a day.

Fruit:  0 0 - Each serving of fruit should be equal to ½ apple or hand full of grapes.

Veg:  0 0 0 0 – choose low in carb vegetables – which most vegetables are except potatoes, yams and sweet potatoes.

Water/ diet drinks – you will need to replace the liquid you lose on this diet.  Drink what you need to replace that and stay hydrated.

Try to think of portion sizes equal to a closed fist and try to remember the pie plate technique – first a protein (a third of your plate), then a vegetable and then a starch.

Fill in the circles as you choose the right foods for weight loss.

Date/Day #7:_____

Protein:  0 0 0 0  - Up to 4 fist sized portions a day.  Fill in each circle as you choose/eat your protein source.

Dairy:  0 0 0 – Milk or cheese – ½-1 cup of milk at each meal or slice of cheese.

Carbs:  0 0 0 – This includes your rice, noodles, pasta and bread.  ½ - 1 cup is enough 1-2 times a day.  Bread – a slice or one bun two times a day.

Fruit:  0 0 - Each serving of fruit should be equal to ½ apple or hand full of grapes.

Veg:  0 0 0 0 – choose low in carb vegetables – which most vegetables are except potatoes, yams and sweet potatoes.

Water/ diet drinks – you will need to replace the liquid you lose on this diet.  Drink what you need to replace that and stay hydrated.

Try to think of portion sizes equal to a closed fist and try to remember the pie plate technique – first a protein (a third of your plate), then a vegetable and then a starch.

Fill in the circles as you choose the right foods for weight loss.

Date/Day #8:_____

Protein:  0 0 0 0  - Up to 4 fist sized portions a day.  Fill in each circle as you choose/eat your protein source.

Dairy: 0 0 0 – Milk or cheese – ½-1 cup of milk at each meal or slice of cheese.

Carbs: 0 0 0 – This includes your rice, noodles, pasta and bread.  ½ - 1 cup is enough 1-2 times a day.  Bread – a slice or one bun two times a day.

Fruit:  0 0 - Each serving of fruit should be equal to ½ apple or hand full of grapes.

Veg:  0 0 0 0 – choose low in carb vegetables – which most vegetables are except potatoes, yams and sweet potatoes.

Water/ diet drinks – you will need to replace the liquid you lose on this diet.  Drink what you need to replace that and stay hydrated.

Try to think of portion sizes equal to a closed fist and try to remember the pie plate technique – first a protein (a third of your plate), then a vegetable and then a starch.

Fill in the circles as you choose the right foods for weight loss.

Date/Day #9:_____

Protein:  0 0 0 0  - Up to 4 fist sized portions a day.  Fill in each circle as you choose/eat your protein source.

Dairy:  0 0 0 – Milk or cheese – ½-1 cup of milk at each meal or slice of cheese.

Carbs:  0 0 0 – This includes your rice, noodles, pasta and bread.  ½ - 1 cup is enough 1-2 times a day.  Bread – a slice or one bun two times a day.

Fruit:  0 0 - Each serving of fruit should be equal to ½ apple or hand full of grapes.

Veg:  0 0 0 0 – choose low in carb vegetables – which most vegetables are except potatoes, yams and sweet potatoes.

Water/ diet drinks – you will need to replace the liquid you lose on this diet.  Drink what you need to replace that and stay hydrated.

Try to think of portion sizes equal to a closed fist and try to remember the pie plate technique – first a protein (a third of your plate), then a vegetable and then a starch.

Fill in the circles as you choose the right foods for weight loss.

Date/Day #10:_____

Protein:  0 0 0 0  - Up to 4 fist sized portions a day.  Fill in each circle as you choose/eat your protein source.

Dairy:  0 0 0 – Milk or cheese – ½-1 cup of milk at each meal or slice of cheese.

Carbs:  0 0 0 – This includes your rice, noodles, pasta and bread.  ½ - 1 cup is enough 1-2 times a day.  Bread – a slice or one bun two times a day.

Fruit:  0 0 - Each serving of fruit should be equal to ½ apple or hand full of grapes.

Veg:  0 0 0 0 – choose low in carb vegetables – which most vegetables are except potatoes, yams and sweet potatoes.

Water/ diet drinks – you will need to replace the liquid you lose on this diet.  Drink what you need to replace that and stay hydrated.

Try to think of portion sizes equal to a closed fist and try to remember the pie plate technique – first a protein (a third of your plate), then a vegetable and then a starch.

Fill in the circles as you choose the right foods for weight loss.

Date/Day #11:_____

Protein:  0 0 0 0  - Up to 4 fist sized portions a day.  Fill in each circle as you choose/eat your protein source.

Dairy:  0 0 0 – Milk or cheese – ½-1 cup of milk at each meal or slice of cheese.

Carbs:  0 0 0 – This includes your rice, noodles, pasta and bread.  ½ - 1 cup is enough 1-2 times a day.  Bread – a slice or one bun two times a day.

Fruit:  0 0 - Each serving of fruit should be equal to ½ apple or hand full of grapes.

Veg:  0 0 0 0 – choose low in carb vegetables – which most vegetables are except potatoes, yams and sweet potatoes.

Water/ diet drinks – you will need to replace the liquid you lose on this diet.  Drink what you need to replace that and stay hydrated.

Try to think of portion sizes equal to a closed fist and try to remember the pie plate technique – first a protein (a third of your plate), then a vegetable and then a starch.

Fill in the circles as you choose the right foods for weight loss.

Date/Day #12:_____

Protein:  0 0 0 0  - Up to 4 fist sized portions a day.  Fill in each circle as you choose/eat your protein source.

Dairy:  0 0 0 – Milk or cheese – ½-1 cup of milk at each meal or slice of cheese.

Carbs:  0 0 0 – This includes your rice, noodles, pasta and bread.  ½ - 1 cup is enough 1-2 times a day.  Bread – a slice or one bun two times a day.

Fruit:  0 0 - Each serving of fruit should be equal to ½ apple or hand full of grapes.

Veg:  0 0 0 0 – choose low in carb vegetables – which most vegetables are except potatoes, yams and sweet potatoes.

Water/ diet drinks – you will need to replace the liquid you lose on this diet.  Drink what you need to replace that and stay hydrated.

Try to think of portion sizes equal to a closed fist and try to remember the pie plate technique – first a protein (a third of your plate), then a vegetable and then a starch.

Fill in the circles as you choose the right foods for weight loss.

Date/Day #13:_____

Protein:  0 0 0 0  - Up to 4 fist sized portions a day.  Fill in each circle as you choose/eat your protein source.

Dairy:  0 0 0 – Milk or cheese – ½-1 cup of milk at each meal or slice of cheese.

Carbs:  0 0 0 – This includes your rice, noodles, pasta and bread.  ½ - 1 cup is enough 1-2 times a day.  Bread – a slice or one bun two times a day.

Fruit:  0 0 - Each serving of fruit should be equal to ½ apple or hand full of grapes.

Veg:  0 0 0 0 – choose low in carb vegetables – which most vegetables are except potatoes, yams and sweet potatoes.

Water/ diet drinks – you will need to replace the liquid you lose on this diet.  Drink what you need to replace that and stay hydrated.

Try to think of portion sizes equal to a closed fist and try to remember the pie plate technique – first a protein (a third of your plate), then a vegetable and then a starch.

Fill in the circles as you choose the right foods for weight loss.

Date/Day #14:_____

Protein:  0 0 0 0  - Up to 4 fist sized portions a day.  Fill in each circle as you choose/eat your protein source.

Dairy:  0 0 0 – Milk or cheese – ½-1 cup of milk at each meal or slice of cheese.

Carbs:  0 0 0 – This includes your rice, noodles, pasta and bread.  ½ - 1 cup is enough 1-2 times a day.  Bread – a slice or one bun two times a day.

Fruit:  0 0 - Each serving of fruit should be equal to ½ apple or hand full of grapes.

Veg:  0 0 0 0 – choose low in carb vegetables – which most vegetables are except potatoes, yams and sweet potatoes.

Water/ diet drinks – you will need to replace the liquid you lose on this diet.  Drink what you need to replace that and stay hydrated.

Try to think of portion sizes equal to a closed fist and try to remember the pie plate technique – first a protein (a third of your plate), then a vegetable and then a starch.

Fill in the circles as you choose the right foods for weight loss.

Date/Day #15:_____

**Protein:** 0 0 0 0 - Up to 4 fist sized portions a day. Fill in each circle as you choose/eat your protein source.

**Dairy:** 0 0 0 – Milk or cheese – ½-1 cup of milk at each meal or slice of cheese.

**Carbs:** 0 0 0 – This includes your rice, noodles, pasta and bread. ½ - 1 cup is enough 1-2 times a day. Bread – a slice or one bun two times a day.

**Fruit:** 0 0 - Each serving of fruit should be equal to ½ apple or hand full of grapes.

**Veg:** 0 0 0 0 – choose low in carb vegetables – which most vegetables are except potatoes, yams and sweet potatoes.

**Water/ diet drinks** – you will need to replace the liquid you lose on this diet. Drink what you need to replace that and stay hydrated.

Try to think of portion sizes equal to a closed fist and try to remember the pie plate technique – first a protein (a third of your plate), then a vegetable and then a starch.

Fill in the circles as you choose the right foods for weight loss.

Date/Day #16:_____

Protein:  0 0 0 0  - Up to 4 fist sized portions a day.  Fill in each circle as you choose/eat your protein source.

Dairy:  0 0 0 – Milk or cheese – ½-1 cup of milk at each meal or slice of cheese.

Carbs:  0 0 0 – This includes your rice, noodles, pasta and bread.  ½ - 1 cup is enough 1-2 times a day.  Bread – a slice or one bun two times a day.

Fruit:  0 0 - Each serving of fruit should be equal to ½ apple or hand full of grapes.

Veg:  0 0 0 0 – choose low in carb vegetables – which most vegetables are except potatoes, yams and sweet potatoes.

Water/ diet drinks – you will need to replace the liquid you lose on this diet.  Drink what you need to replace that and stay hydrated.

Try to think of portion sizes equal to a closed fist and try to remember the pie plate technique – first a protein (a third of your plate), then a vegetable and then a starch.

Fill in the circles as you choose the right foods for weight loss.

Date/Day #17:_____

Protein:  0 0 0 0  - Up to 4 fist sized portions a day.  Fill in each circle as you choose/eat your protein source.

Dairy:  0 0 0 – Milk or cheese – ½-1 cup of milk at each meal or slice of cheese.

Carbs:  0 0 0 – This includes your rice, noodles, pasta and bread.  ½ - 1 cup is enough 1-2 times a day.  Bread – a slice or one bun two times a day.

Fruit:  0 0 - Each serving of fruit should be equal to ½ apple or hand full of grapes.

Veg:  0 0 0 0 – choose low in carb vegetables – which most vegetables are except potatoes, yams and sweet potatoes.

Water/ diet drinks – you will need to replace the liquid you lose on this diet.  Drink what you need to replace that and stay hydrated.

Try to think of portion sizes equal to a closed fist and try to remember the pie plate technique – first a protein (a third of your plate), then a vegetable and then a starch.

Fill in the circles as you choose the right foods for weight loss.

Date/Day #18:_____

Protein: 0 0 0 0 - Up to 4 fist sized portions a day. Fill in each circle as you choose/eat your protein source.

Dairy: 0 0 0 – Milk or cheese – ½-1 cup of milk at each meal or slice of cheese.

Carbs: 0 0 0 – This includes your rice, noodles, pasta and bread. ½ - 1 cup is enough 1-2 times a day. Bread – a slice or one bun two times a day.

Fruit: 0 0 - Each serving of fruit should be equal to ½ apple or hand full of grapes.

Veg: 0 0 0 0 – choose low in carb vegetables – which most vegetables are except potatoes, yams and sweet potatoes.

Water/ diet drinks – you will need to replace the liquid you lose on this diet. Drink what you need to replace that and stay hydrated.

Try to think of portion sizes equal to a closed fist and try to remember the pie plate technique – first a protein (a third of your plate), then a vegetable and then a starch.

Fill in the circles as you choose the right foods for weight loss.

Date/Day #19:_____

Protein:  0 0 0 0  - Up to 4 fist sized portions a day.  Fill in each circle as you choose/eat your protein source.

Dairy:  0 0 0 – Milk or cheese – ½-1 cup of milk at each meal or slice of cheese.

Carbs:  0 0 0 – This includes your rice, noodles, pasta and bread.  ½ - 1 cup is enough 1-2 times a day.  Bread – a slice or one bun two times a day.

Fruit:  0 0 - Each serving of fruit should be equal to ½ apple or hand full of grapes.

Veg:  0 0 0 0 – choose low in carb vegetables – which most vegetables are except potatoes, yams and sweet potatoes.

Water/ diet drinks – you will need to replace the liquid you lose on this diet.  Drink what you need to replace that and stay hydrated.

Try to think of portion sizes equal to a closed fist and try to remember the pie plate technique – first a protein (a third of your plate), then a vegetable and then a starch.

Fill in the circles as you choose the right foods for weight loss.

Date/Day #20:_____

Protein:  0 0 0 0  - Up to 4 fist sized portions a day.  Fill in each circle as you choose/eat your protein source.

Dairy:  0 0 0 – Milk or cheese – ½-1 cup of milk at each meal or slice of cheese.

Carbs:  0 0 0 – This includes your rice, noodles, pasta and bread.  ½ - 1 cup is enough 1-2 times a day.  Bread – a slice or one bun two times a day.

Fruit:  0 0 - Each serving of fruit should be equal to ½ apple or hand full of grapes.

Veg:  0 0 0 0 – choose low in carb vegetables – which most vegetables are except potatoes, yams and sweet potatoes.

Water/ diet drinks – you will need to replace the liquid you lose on this diet.  Drink what you need to replace that and stay hydrated.

Try to think of portion sizes equal to a closed fist and try to remember the pie plate technique – first a protein (a third of your plate), then a vegetable and then a starch.

Fill in the circles as you choose the right foods for weight loss.

Date/Day #21:_____

**Protein:  0 0 0 0**  - Up to 4 fist sized portions a day.  Fill in each circle as you choose/eat your protein source.

**Dairy:  0 0 0** – Milk or cheese – ½-1 cup of milk at each meal or slice of cheese.

**Carbs:  0 0 0** – This includes your rice, noodles, pasta and bread.  ½ - 1 cup is enough 1-2 times a day.  Bread – a slice or one bun two times a day.

**Fruit:  0 0** - Each serving of fruit should be equal to ½ apple or hand full of grapes.

**Veg:  0 0 0 0** – choose low in carb vegetables – which most vegetables are except potatoes, yams and sweet potatoes.

**Water/ diet drinks** – you will need to replace the liquid you lose on this diet.  Drink what you need to replace that and stay hydrated.

Try to think of portion sizes equal to a closed fist and try to remember the pie plate technique – first a protein (a third of your plate), then a vegetable and then a starch.

Fill in the circles as you choose the right foods for weight loss.

Date/Day #22:_____

Protein:  0 0 0 0  - Up to 4 fist sized portions a day.  Fill in each circle as you choose/eat your protein source.

Dairy:  0 0 0 – Milk or cheese – ½-1 cup of milk at each meal or slice of cheese.

Carbs:  0 0 0 – This includes your rice, noodles, pasta and bread.  ½ - 1 cup is enough 1-2 times a day.  Bread – a slice or one bun two times a day.

Fruit:  0 0 - Each serving of fruit should be equal to ½ apple or hand full of grapes.

Veg:  0 0 0 0 – choose low in carb vegetables – which most vegetables are except potatoes, yams and sweet potatoes.

Water/ diet drinks – you will need to replace the liquid you lose on this diet.  Drink what you need to replace that and stay hydrated.

Try to think of portion sizes equal to a closed fist and try to remember the pie plate technique – first a protein (a third of your plate), then a vegetable and then a starch.

Fill in the circles as you choose the right foods for weight loss.

Date/Day #23:_____

Protein:  0 0 0 0  - Up to 4 fist sized portions a day.  Fill in each circle as you choose/eat your protein source.

Dairy:  0 0 0 – Milk or cheese – ½-1 cup of milk at each meal or slice of cheese.

Carbs:  0 0 0 – This includes your rice, noodles, pasta and bread.  ½ - 1 cup is enough 1-2 times a day.  Bread – a slice or one bun two times a day.

Fruit:  0 0 - Each serving of fruit should be equal to ½ apple or hand full of grapes.

Veg:  0 0 0 0 – choose low in carb vegetables – which most vegetables are except potatoes, yams and sweet potatoes.

Water/ diet drinks – you will need to replace the liquid you lose on this diet.  Drink what you need to replace that and stay hydrated.

Try to think of portion sizes equal to a closed fist and try to remember the pie plate technique – first a protein (a third of your plate), then a vegetable and then a starch.

Fill in the circles as you choose the right foods for weight loss.

Date/Day #24:_____

Protein:  0 0 0 0  - Up to 4 fist sized portions a day.  Fill in each circle as you choose/eat your protein source.

Dairy:  0 0 0 – Milk or cheese – ½-1 cup of milk at each meal or slice of cheese.

Carbs:  0 0 0 – This includes your rice, noodles, pasta and bread.  ½ - 1 cup is enough 1-2 times a day.  Bread – a slice or one bun two times a day.

Fruit:  0 0 - Each serving of fruit should be equal to ½ apple or hand full of grapes.

Veg:  0 0 0 0 – choose low in carb vegetables – which most vegetables are except potatoes, yams and sweet potatoes.

Water/ diet drinks – you will need to replace the liquid you lose on this diet.  Drink what you need to replace that and stay hydrated.

Try to think of portion sizes equal to a closed fist and try to remember the pie plate technique – first a protein (a third of your plate), then a vegetable and then a starch.

Fill in the circles as you choose the right foods for weight loss.

Date/Day #25:_____

Protein:  0 0 0 0  - Up to 4 fist sized portions a day.  Fill in each circle as you choose/eat your protein source.

Dairy:  0 0 0 – Milk or cheese – ½-1 cup of milk at each meal or slice of cheese.

Carbs:  0 0 0 – This includes your rice, noodles, pasta and bread.  ½ - 1 cup is enough 1-2 times a day.  Bread – a slice or one bun two times a day.

Fruit:  0 0 - Each serving of fruit should be equal to ½ apple or hand full of grapes.

Veg:  0 0 0 0 – choose low in carb vegetables – which most vegetables are except potatoes, yams and sweet potatoes.

Water/ diet drinks – you will need to replace the liquid you lose on this diet.  Drink what you need to replace that and stay hydrated.

Try to think of portion sizes equal to a closed fist and try to remember the pie plate technique – first a protein (a third of your plate), then a vegetable and then a starch.

Fill in the circles as you choose the right foods for weight loss.

Date/Day #26:_____

Protein:  0 0 0 0  - Up to 4 fist sized portions a day.  Fill in each circle as you choose/eat your protein source.

Dairy:  0 0 0 – Milk or cheese – ½-1 cup of milk at each meal or slice of cheese.

Carbs:  0 0 0 – This includes your rice, noodles, pasta and bread.  ½ - 1 cup is enough 1-2 times a day.  Bread – a slice or one bun two times a day.

Fruit:  0 0 - Each serving of fruit should be equal to ½ apple or hand full of grapes.

Veg:  0 0 0 0 – choose low in carb vegetables – which most vegetables are except potatoes, yams and sweet potatoes.

Water/ diet drinks – you will need to replace the liquid you lose on this diet.  Drink what you need to replace that and stay hydrated.

Try to think of portion sizes equal to a closed fist and try to remember the pie plate technique – first a protein (a third of your plate), then a vegetable and then a starch.

Fill in the circles as you choose the right foods for weight loss.

Date/Day #27:_____

**Protein:  0 0 0 0** - Up to 4 fist sized portions a day.  Fill in each circle as you choose/eat your protein source.

**Dairy:  0 0 0** – Milk or cheese – ½-1 cup of milk at each meal or slice of cheese.

**Carbs:  0 0 0** – This includes your rice, noodles, pasta and bread.  ½ - 1 cup is enough 1-2 times a day.  Bread – a slice or one bun two times a day.

**Fruit:  0 0** - Each serving of fruit should be equal to ½ apple or hand full of grapes.

**Veg:  0 0 0 0** – choose low in carb vegetables – which most vegetables are except potatoes, yams and sweet potatoes.

**Water/ diet drinks** – you will need to replace the liquid you lose on this diet.  Drink what you need to replace that and stay hydrated.

Try to think of portion sizes equal to a closed fist and try to remember the pie plate technique – first a protein (a third of your plate), then a vegetable and then a starch.

Fill in the circles as you choose the right foods for weight loss.

Date/Day #28:_____

Protein:  0 0 0 0  - Up to 4 fist sized portions a day.  Fill in each circle as you choose/eat your protein source.

Dairy:  0 0 0 – Milk or cheese – ½-1 cup of milk at each meal or slice of cheese.

Carbs:  0 0 0 – This includes your rice, noodles, pasta and bread.  ½ - 1 cup is enough 1-2 times a day.  Bread – a slice or one bun two times a day.

Fruit:  0 0 - Each serving of fruit should be equal to ½ apple or hand full of grapes.

Veg:  0 0 0 0 – choose low in carb vegetables – which most vegetables are except potatoes, yams and sweet potatoes.

Water/ diet drinks – you will need to replace the liquid you lose on this diet.  Drink what you need to replace that and stay hydrated.

Try to think of portion sizes equal to a closed fist and try to remember the pie plate technique – first a protein (a third of your plate), then a vegetable and then a starch.

Fill in the circles as you choose the right foods for weight loss.

Date/Day #29:_____

Protein:  0 0 0 0  - Up to 4 fist sized portions a day.  Fill in each circle as you choose/eat your protein source.

Dairy:  0 0 0 – Milk or cheese – ½-1 cup of milk at each meal or slice of cheese.

Carbs:  0 0 0 – This includes your rice, noodles, pasta and bread.  ½ - 1 cup is enough 1-2 times a day.  Bread – a slice or one bun two times a day.

Fruit:  0 0 - Each serving of fruit should be equal to ½ apple or hand full of grapes.

Veg:  0 0 0 0 – choose low in carb vegetables – which most vegetables are except potatoes, yams and sweet potatoes.

Water/ diet drinks – you will need to replace the liquid you lose on this diet.  Drink what you need to replace that and stay hydrated.

Try to think of portion sizes equal to a closed fist and try to remember the pie plate technique – first a protein (a third of your plate), then a vegetable and then a starch.

Fill in the circles as you choose the right foods for weight loss.

Date/Day #30:_____

Protein:  0 0 0 0  - Up to 4 fist sized portions a day.  Fill in each circle as you choose/eat your protein source.

Dairy:  0 0 0 – Milk or cheese – ½-1 cup of milk at each meal or slice of cheese.

Carbs:  0 0 0 – This includes your rice, noodles, pasta and bread.  ½ - 1 cup is enough 1-2 times a day.  Bread – a slice or one bun two times a day.

Fruit:  0 0 - Each serving of fruit should be equal to ½ apple or hand full of grapes.

Veg:  0 0 0 0 – choose low in carb vegetables – which most vegetables are except potatoes, yams and sweet potatoes.

Water/ diet drinks – you will need to replace the liquid you lose on this diet.  Drink what you need to replace that and stay hydrated.

Try to think of portion sizes equal to a closed fist and try to remember the pie plate technique – first a protein (a third of your plate), then a vegetable and then a starch.

Fill in the circles as you choose the right foods for weight loss.